Pharmacological Effects of Zingiber Officinale Extract in Rodents

Cytoprotective Effect of Zingiber Officinale Extract On Alcohol Induced Gastric Lesion in Mice

Samia Elzwi
Amina Elzwi

ELIVA PRESS

ELIVA PRESS

Samia Elzwi

Amina Elzwi

Ginger is a perennial plant that grows in India, China, Mexico and several other countries. The rhizome is used as both spice and in herbal medicine. Many studies have been done on pharmacological effect of ginger extract and our paper has been focused on cytoprotective effect of ginger on ethanol induced gastric injury in mice. Many drugs have been used in the treatment of peptic ulcer but each of them associated with different side effect so trends today toward use of herbal medicine which was associated with adverse effect. Ginger hydroalcoholic extract contain different consistent with anti-ulcer properties like 6-Gingersulfonic acid and three monoacyldigalactosyl glycerol including ginger glycolipid A. B. C. The mechanism of ginger extract may be due to counteracting the active oxidant radicals, decreasing mucosal cell shedding and thicking the mucus membrane so ginger extract has antiulcer properties when used in accurate dose and accurate duration.

Published by Eliva Press SRL
Address: MD-2060, bd.Cuza-Voda, 1/4, of. 21 Chişinău, Republica
Moldova
Email: info@elivapress.com
Website: www.elivapress.com

ISBN: 978-1-63648-107-4

Pharmacological Effects of Zingiber Officinale Extract in Rodents

Samia Elzwi[1] and Amina Elzwi[2]

1.MSc Assistant professor at pharmacology department, University of Benghazi, Libya

2.Pharmacy doctor at faculty of pharmacy, University of Benghazi, Libya

Table of contents:

List of figures

Pharmacological Effects of Zingiber Officinale Extract in Rodents

Samia Elzwi[1] and Amina Elzwi[2]

1.MSc Assistant professor at pharmacology department, University of Benghazi, Libya

2.Pharmacy doctor at faculty of pharmacy, University of Benghazi, Libya

Abstract: Ginger is a perennial plant that grows in India, China, Mexico and several other countries. The rhizome is used as both spice and in herbal medicine. Many studies have been done on pharmacological effect of ginger extract and our paper has been focused on cytoprotective effect of ginger on ethanol induced gastric injury in mice. Many drugs have been used in the treatment of peptic ulcer but each of them associated with different side effect so trends today toward use of herbal medicine which was associated with adverse effect. Ginger hydroalcoholic extract contain different consistent with anti-ulcer properties like 6-Gingersulfonic acid and three monoacyldigalactosyl glycerol including ginger glycolipid A. B. C .The mechanism of ginger extract may be due to counteracting the active oxidant radicals, decreasing mucosal cell shedding and thicking the mucus membrane so ginger extract has antiulcer properties when used in accurate dose and accurate duration.

(Zingiber officinale) ginger has hepatoprotective effect through antioxidant properties.

Keywords: Acetaminophen Cytoprotective effect, Ethanol, Ginger hydroalcoholic extract, Mice, Zingiber Officinale, Hepatotoxicity, Hepatoprotective effect.

Introduction: Spices, the predominant flavoring, coloring, and aromatic agents in food and beverages are now gaining importance for their diversified uses. Ginger (Zingiber Officinale) is a medicinal plant that has been widely used in Chinese, and Tibb Unani herbal medicines all over the world, since antiquity, for a wide array of unrelated ailments that include muscular aches, sore throat, constipation, arthritis,

3

indigestion, vomiting and infectious diseases. Currently, there is a renewed interest in ginger, and several scientific investigations aimed at isolation and identification of active constituents of ginger, scientific verification of its pharmacological actions and of its constituents, and verification of the basis of the use of ginger in several diseases and conditions(Ali et al 2007). Ginger grows best in tropical and subtropical areas, which have good rainfall with hot and humid conditions during the summer season. It is a member of Zingiberaceae family originated in Southeast Asia and has been introduced to many parts of the globe where it proliferates in suitable environment. Belief in the medicinal properties of ginger existed in ancient Indian and oriental cultures where ginger has been used alone or as a component in herbal remedies. This practice continues today in many areas of the world including Africa, Brazil, China and, Mexico. Ginger has introduced to Europe and other areas by Dutch, Portuguese Arab and Spanish explorers or traders from around the 13th to 16th centuries.

Consitutents. 1.Carbohydrates: starch is major constituents up to 50%.

2. Oleo-resin: gingerol homologues (major, about 33%) include derivatives with methyl side chain, shogaol homologues (dehydration products of gingerols), zingerone (degradation product of gingerols) , 1- dehydrogingerdione and 6-gingersulfonic acid.

3. Lipids 6-8%: They include free fatty acids e.g palmitic acid, oleic acid, linoleic acid, caprylic acid, capric acid, lauric acid, myristic acid, pentadecanoic acid, heptadecanoic acid, stearic acid, linolenic acid, arachidonic acid ,triglycerides, phosphatidic acid, lecithins and gingerglycolipids A, B and C3.

4. Volatile oil: They constitute 1-3% they are complex predominately Hydrocarbons, zingiberene (major components) and B-bisabolene. Other sesquiterpenes include zingiberol, zingiberenol. 5. Other constitutes: Include amino acids as arginine, aspartic acid, cystine, glycine, isoleucine, leucine, serine, threonine and valine. Proteins constitute about 9%

Diterpenes (galanolactone), vitamins especially nicotinic acid (niacin) and vitamin A as well as minerals are also present.

Description: The common cooking ginger is an herbaceous perennial plant with upright stems and narrow medium green leaves arranged in two ranks on each stem. The plant gets about 1.2cm tall with leaves and 1.9 cm wide and 17.8 cm long. Ginger grows from an aromatic tubelike rhizome (underground stem) which is warty and branched.

The inflorescence grows on separate stem from the foliage stem and forms a dense spike 7.6 cm tall. The barcts are green with translucent margins and the small flowers are yellow green with purple lips and cream-colored blotches.

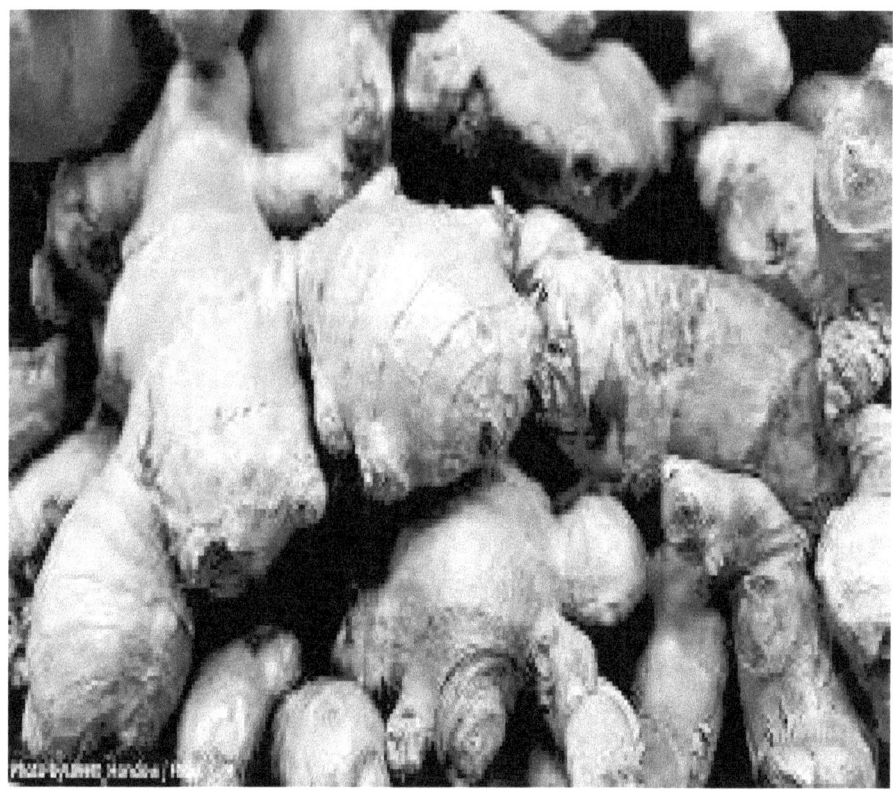

Figure (1): Fresh ginger rhizome

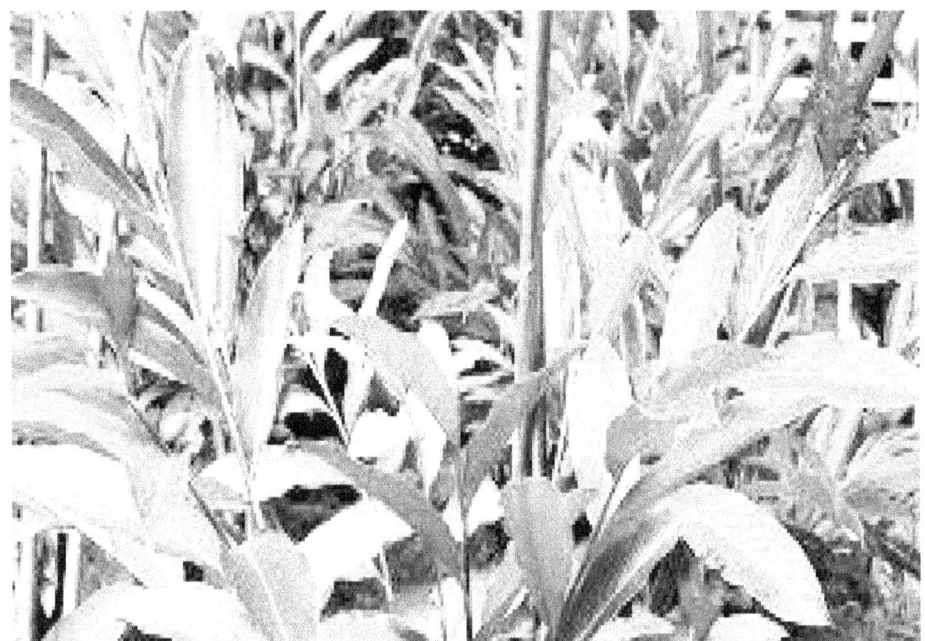

Figure (2): Ginger plant leaves

Table (1): Scientific classification of Ginger

kingdom………………Plantae

phylum…………………Tracheophyta

class…………………..Liliopsida

order…………………… Zingiberales

family…………………..Zingiberaceae

species……………….. Zingiber officinale

Pharmacokinetics: After injection 90% of 6-gingerol is bound to serum protein and elimination mainly via the liver. Oral or intraperitoneal dosage of zingerone results in urinary excretion of metabolites within 24 hours mainly as glucuronide and sulphate conjugation Appreciable biliary excretion 40% occurs in 12 hours

Cytoprotective Effect of Zingiber Officinale Extract on Alcohol Induced Gastric Lesion in Mice

Ulcer are caused due to imbalance between aggressive factors (hydrochloric acid, pepsin, gastrin, no steroidal anti-inflammatory drugs, and ethanol) and defensive factor of gastric mucosa (prostaglandin, mucus, bicarbonate). The antiulcerogenic activity of many plant products is reported due to an increase in mucosal defensive factors rather than decrease in the aggressive factors(Goel, et al 1985). Numbers of an antiulcer drugs like gastric antisecretory drugs H2- receptor antagonist, antimuscarinic agents, proton pump inhibitors, and mucosal protective agents, carbenoxolone sodium, sucralfate, and prostaglandin analogous are available which are shown to have side effects and limitation(Baowman et al , 1982)

8

There are several herbal ayuvedic preparation which have a protective effect against gastric mucosal injury (Shetty et al 2000). Herbal medicine is now used by up to 50% of the Western population in a number of instances 10% for treatment or prevention of digestive disorders (Langmead and Rampton,2001)Today, pharmacopoeias of a number of different countries list ginger extract for various digestive disease, Aromatic, spasmolytic and carminative properties of ginger are probably responsible for the therapeutic application in digestive tract ailments (Sertie et al.1992)

Mechanism of Gastric Effect of Ginger: Several studies have shown that ginger extract, essential oils and glycolipids possess a number of pharmacological actions, which at least in part for some of them anti-ulcerogenic or ulcer preventive efficacy may be suggested. Common side effects of treating inflammation with modern drugs is that ulcer in the digestive system can be created or their condition made worse (Wallace, 1996). Ginger not only relieves the symptoms of inflammation but also protects the creation of digestive ulcers. Ginger may protect the stomach from the damaging effect of alcohol and non- steroidal anti-inflammatory drugs and may help prevent ulcers(Villegas et al. 2004) .A study was done in Isfahan university by (Miniaiyan et al 2006.) for anti-ulcerogenic effect of ginger on cysteamine-induced duodenal ulcer in rats. The results obtained in positive control groups indicated that ginger possesses its anti-ulcerative properties through a mechanism mainly related to acid- pepsin inhibition. The effect of ginger (acetone extract) and zingiberene on hydrochlochloric acid/ethanol-induced gastric lesions in rats have been examined (6)- gingerol and zingiberene, both 100mg/ kg oral), significantly inhibited gastric lesions by 54.5% and 53.6% respectively. The total extract inhibited lesions by 97.5% at 1g/kg. Oral administration of both aqueous and methanol ginger extract to rabbit has been reported to reduce gastric secretions (gastric juice volume, acid and pepsin output). Both extracts were found to be comparable with cimetidine (50mg/kg) with respect to gastric juice volume. The aqueous extract was comparable with cimetidine and superior to the methanol extract for pepsin output, and the methanol extract to cimetidine for acid output. superior to the aqueous extract and comparable

Roasted ginger decoction which showed an obvious inhibiting tendency on three gastric ulcer models. The plant contains active materials which for some of them ulcer protective properties have been identified 6- ginger sulfonic acid and three monoacyldigalactosyl glycerols including ginger glycolipid A,B,C have been isolated from dried rhizome of Zingiber Officinale which are potent anti-ulcer components (Yoshikawa et al 1992)..a) 6- gingerol and 6- shagaol are two other anti-ulcer components that are less potent but responsible for ginger pungency.

b). Results of one study fore effects of three herbal medicine including Zingiber Officinale on gastric ulceration and secretion in rats indicated significant protection against stress, aspirin and pylorus ligation. The proposed anti-ulcerogenic effects were augmentation of mucin secretion and decrease in cell shedding.

c) (Al-Yahya et al 1989). Studied the cytoprotective and gastric anti-ulcer effect of ginger in albino rats. Cyto destruction was produced by 80% ethanol, 0.6M HCL, 0.2 M NaOH and 25% Nacl. Gastric ulcer was produced by ulcerogenic agents including indomethacin, aspirin and reserpine beside hypothermic restraint stress and by pylorus ligation. The results of this study demonstrated that the extract in the dose 500mg/kg orally exerted highly significant cryoprotection and prevented occurrence of gastric ulcer induced by non-steroidal anti-inflammatory drugs.

METHODOLOGY A. Experimental animals: Albino mice of either sex weighing 20-30 g, and male Wistar strain rats, weighing 200-250 g were maintained in the animal house of Faculty of Medicine – Al Arab Medical University, The mice and rat were rats were bred in the faculty animal house. All animals were housed in standard polypropylene cages(48×35×22cm) Benghazi, Libya and kept under controlled room temperature (20±5 ◦C; relative humidity 60-70%) in a 12 h light-dark cycle. The animals were given a standard laboratory diet and free water. Food was withdrawn 12 .h before and during the experimental hours

B. Preparation of Zingiber officinale extract: Maceration method: In this method fresh ginger rhizome was cut into small pieces, dried, and then pulverized into coarse powder and weighing about400 g of powder. It was macerated in 1000 ml hydroalcoholic solution (70% Ethanol, 30% distilled water) for seventy-two hours the extract was then shaken, filtered by using filter paper and the solution was evaporated in a rotatory evaporator under reduced pressure until dryness. Evaporation and removal of the solvent give hydroalcoholic extract of ginger out of 400g of crude plant, 8g of hydroalcoholic extract of ginger were obtained and kept for use in pharmacological experiments (Iranian Herbal Pharmacopeia).

Study of cytoprotective effect of hydroalcoholic extract of ginger in an animal model of gastric lesion. Mice of either sex weighing 25-30g were employed in this study the animals were divided into six groups each consisting of six mice.

1. Normal group: Given vehicle (5ml/kg orally) without ulcer induction.

2. Control group: Given vehicle (5ml/kg orally) one hour before ulcer induction.

3. Extract group: Given hydroalcoholic extract of ginger in a dose (300mg/kg orally) one hour before ulcer induction.

4. Extract group: Given hydroalcoholic extract of ginger in a dose of (600mg/kg I.P) one hour before ulcer induction.

5. Chronic extract group: Given hydroalcoholic extract of ginger. In a dose of (300mg/kg I.P) for five consecutive days before ulcer induction. The last dose was administered one hour before ulcer induction.

6. Reference group: Given ranitidine (50mg/kg I.P) one hour before ulcer induction. One hour after intragastric administration of absolute ethanol (95%, 0.2ml), the animals are euthanized with ether, the stomach were excised, cut along the greater curvature, and gently rinsed under tap water, and examined by 5 fold binocular magnifier to assess lesion in gastric mucosa.

 Results: As shown in Figure (3) normal gastric mucosa compared with Figure (4&5) with treatment by ethanol there is exfoliation and sloughing of gastric cells with inflammatory cell infiltrate and congestion of blood vessels Figure (6). Figure

(7)shows partial improvement in gastric lesion in the group treated by oral ginger treatment at dose 300mg/kg as there is mild exfoliation of gastric cells Figure (7) .Moderate gastric protection by (I.P) treatment of ginger at a dose 600mg/kg as there is moderate exfoliation of gastric cells as shown in Figure (8) .Complete protection by chronic (I.P) treatment of ginger in a dose of 300mg/kg with no exfoliation of gastric cells as shown in Figure (9). Ranitidine has moderate protective effect as shown in Figure (10).

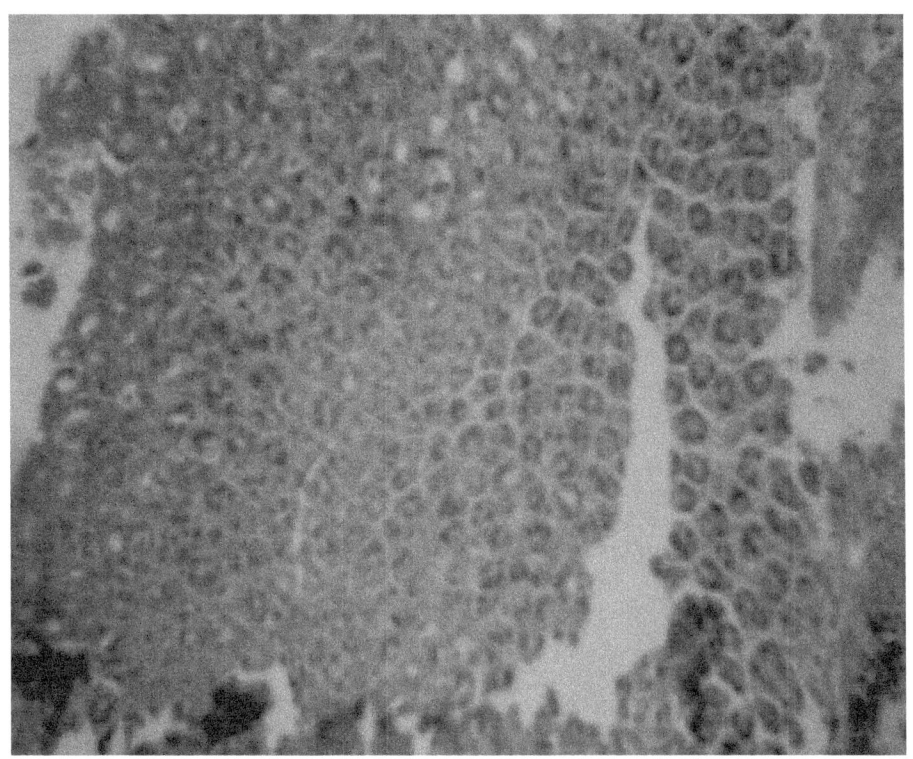

Figure (3) : Normal gastrc mucosa

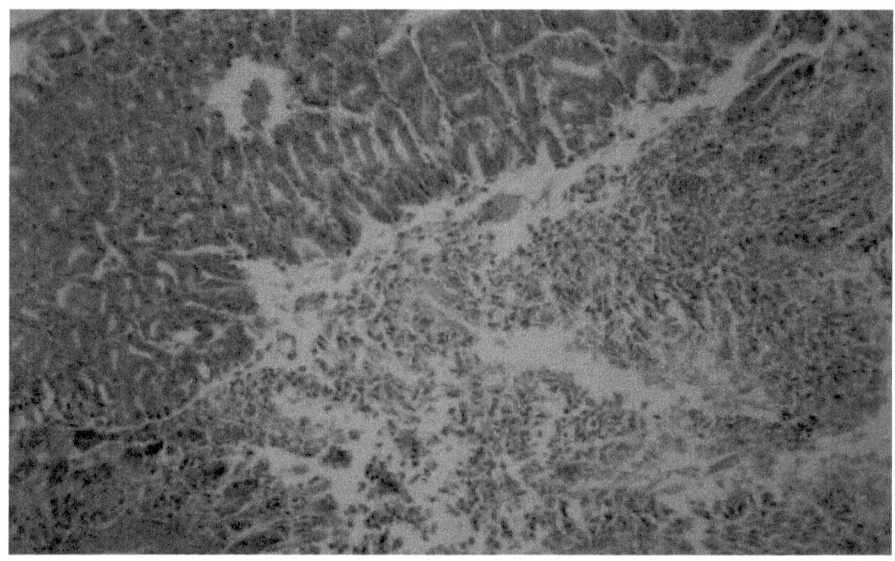

Figure 4 : Ethanol treated mucosa with exfoliation and sloughing-

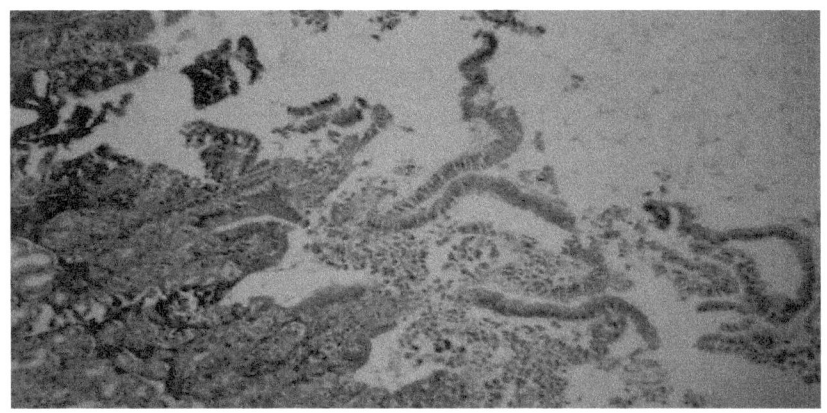

Figure (5): Ethanol treated stomach with exfolition and sloughing

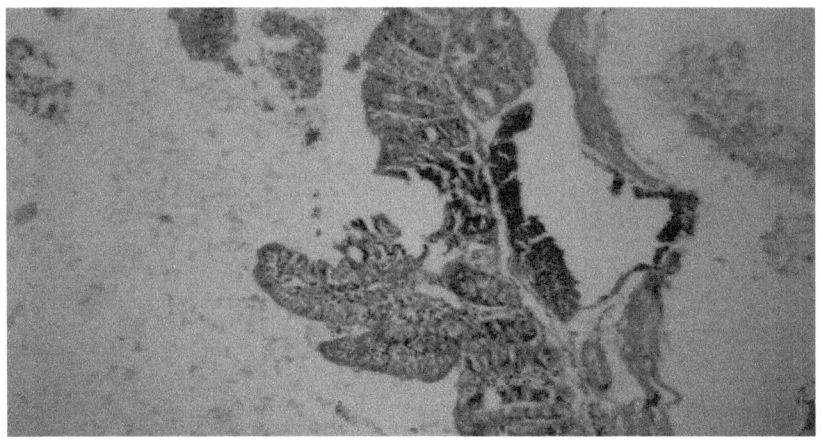

Figure (6): Ethanol treated stomach with congestion of blood vessels

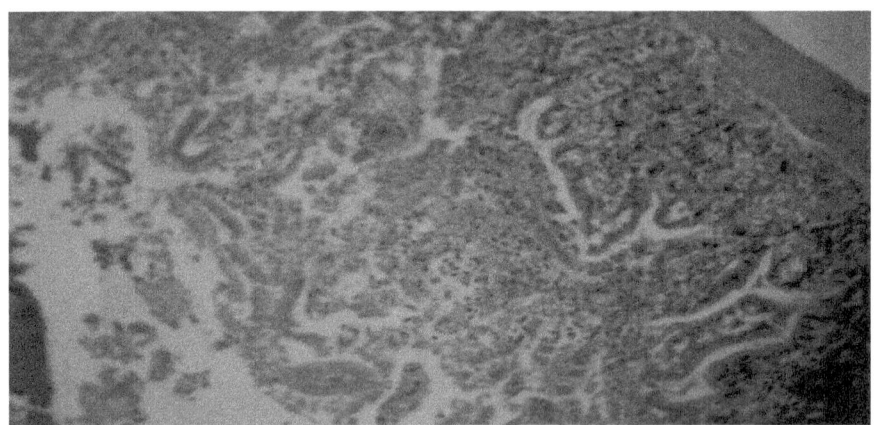

Figure (7) : Ginger treated stomach (p.o)

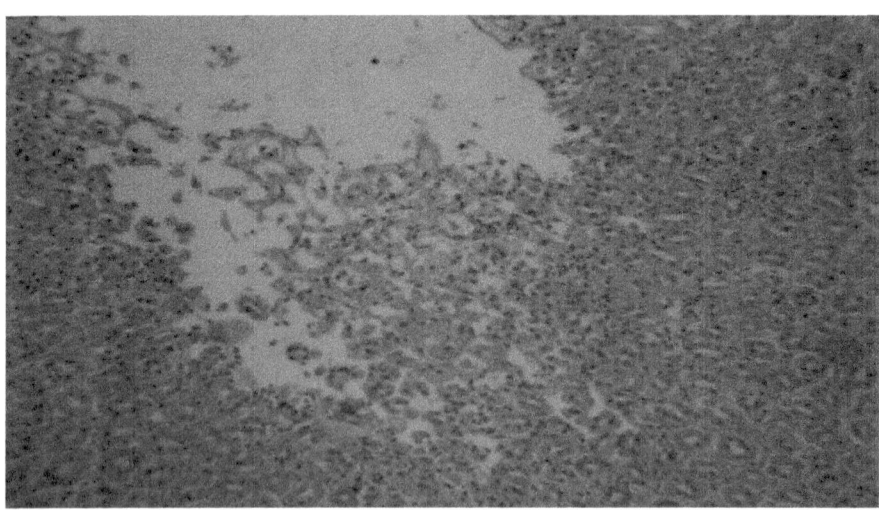

Figure (8) : Ginger treated stomach (i.p)

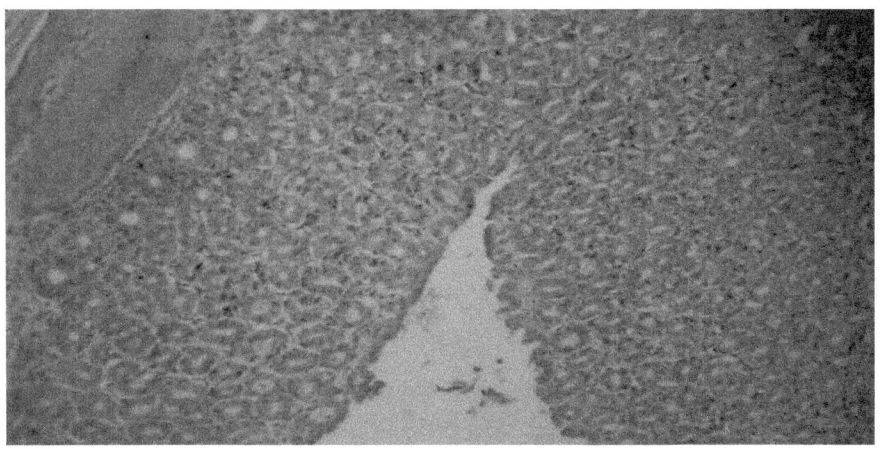

Figure (9) : Chronic ginger treated stomach (i.p)

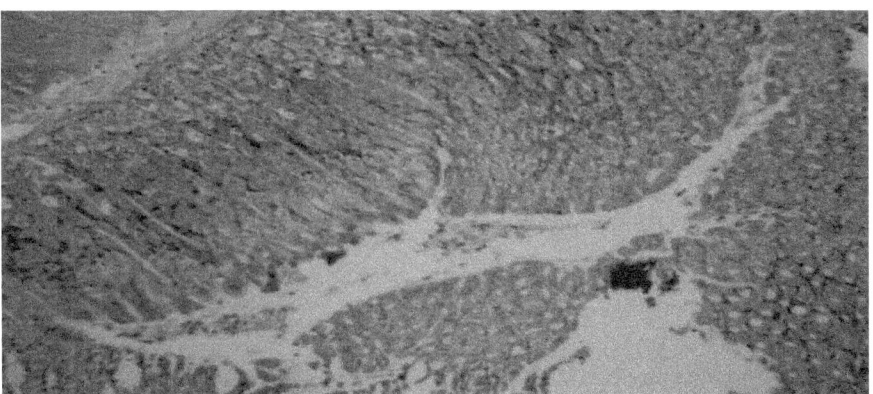

Figure (10) : Ranitidine treated stomach (i.p)

Discussion: The mucosal injuries as evidence by necrosis, exfoliation and sloughing of gastric cells, congestion of blood vessels and infiltration of inflammatory cells. Cytoprotective action of ginger has been investigated using animal models of acute gastric injury induced by necrotizing agents such as ethanol. Ethanol serves as the most common ulcerogenic agent and produced sever gastric hemorrhagic erosions (Robert et al 1979). ;Szabo et al 1981). The genesis of ethanol-induced gastric lesions is multifactorial with the depletion of gastric wall mucus content as one of the involved factors. Submucosal venular constriction by ethanol and eventual injury is caused due to perturbations of superficial mucosal cells, notably the mucosal mast cells leading to release of vasoactive mediators including histamine, that cause damage to gastric mucosa (Hollander et al.1984) .Accumulation of activated neutrophil in gastric mucosa may be the source of free radicals Oxygen free radical which lead to increase to lipid peroxidation and damage to cell membrane are impacted in ethanol induced gastric mucosal injury (Al-Harbi et al1997). In addition to its direct damage of gastric mucosal cells by development of free radicals, cause solubilization of mucus constituents and depressant tissue levels of protein leading to flow stasis in gastric blood. The present paper revealed partial cryoprotection by single oral dose of ginger (300mg/kg) in mice more effective cytoprotection was elicited by ginger in dose (600mg/kg i.p).

The result obtained in the present paper indicated that ginger extract possess its antiulcer properties through mechanism mainly related to acid and pepsin inhibition Chronic I.P injection of plant extract in a dose of (300mg/kg) more effective in prevention lesion formation. The mechanism of ginger extract in chronic (I.P) protection may be due to counteracting the active oxidant radicals, decreasing mucosal cell shedding and thicking the mucus membrane. The mechanism of anti-ulcer effect of ginger may be due to presence of 6-Gingersulfonic acid and three monoacyldigalactosyl gylcerols including ginger glycolipid A. B. C have been isolated from dried rhizome of Zingiber Officinale which are potent anti-ulcer components (Yoshikawa et al. 1992) 6- Gingerol and 6- shogaol are two other anti-ulcer components that are less potent but are mainly responsible for ginger pungency. The results of present paper in accordance with previous reports in which water and methanolic extract of eight Zingiberaceae herbs caused a significant decrease in gastric secretion in un-anesthetized rabbits and the effect of water extract was similar to cimetidine (sakai et al., 1989).

Effect of Zingiber officinale (Ginger) Extract on Acetaminophen Induced Hepatotoxicity in Mice

In this experiment mice of either sex weighing 25-30g were divided into three groups, each consisting of seven mice. The animals were fasted for twelve hours prior to the experiment with free access to water.

1.Control group: Given normal saline containing 0.5 % Tween-80 (orally) in a dose of 1ml each mice

2. Extract group: Given hydroalcoholic extract of ginger in a dose of (300mg/kg ip) for 14 days followed by acetaminophen (300mg/kg i.p) on the 15th day from starting of the extract.

3. Acetaminophen group: Given acetaminophen in single (i.p) injection of 300mg/kg. By the end of 24hr following the injection of acetaminophen, the number of deaths in each group was calculated, all animals were fasted for18 hrs. Before sacrifice. The collected blood used for measurement of liver transaminases and the livers were isolated, fixed in 10% formalin for histopathological analysis

RESULTS: Compared to the control group that showed no death of animals, the acetaminophen treated group showed 2 deaths out of seven mice. This was reduced to 1 death of seven in the Zingiber officinal+ acetaminophen treated group.6 As present in this figure the levels of AST where 142± 8.95, 90.66±16.54, 471±80.84 unit/ml in control, Zingiber officinale+ acetaminophen and acetaminophen treated group, whereas the level of ALT was 57.2±4.61, 31.66±9.36, 402±105.19 unit/ml in animal receiving the previously mentioned treatment respectively. By using one-way ANOV and Post Hoc analysis, the level of AST and ALT was higher in acetaminophen treated group compared to the other group p≤ 0.00. The statistical analysis showed that the levels of AST and ALT in the Zingiber officinale + acetaminophen treated group were not significantly changed compared with control group.7 Histological studies also provided evidence for the biochemical analysis. The control and Zingiber officinale treated groups showed the normal hepatocytes, portal tracts and central vein (Figure 11). Centrizonal necrosis accompanied by fatty changes were observed in the hepatocytes in the livers of mice in acetaminophen treated group (Figure12, 13). The cellular necrosis was almost completely disappearing in the group treated with Zingiber officinale + acetaminophen groups (Figure 14).

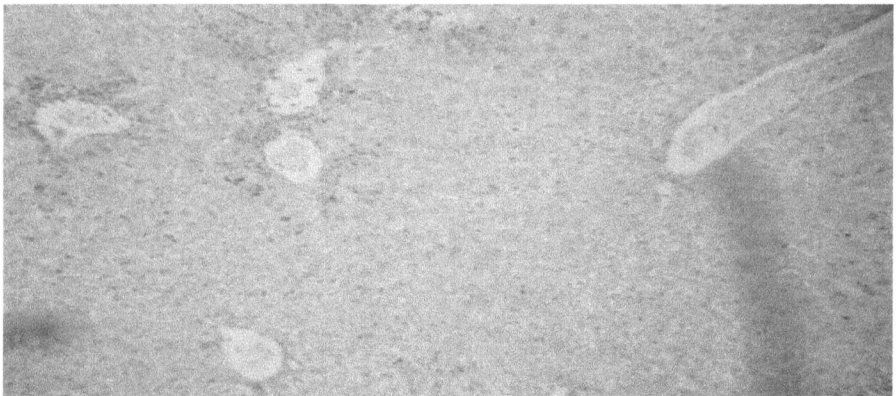

Figure (11) : Normal liver

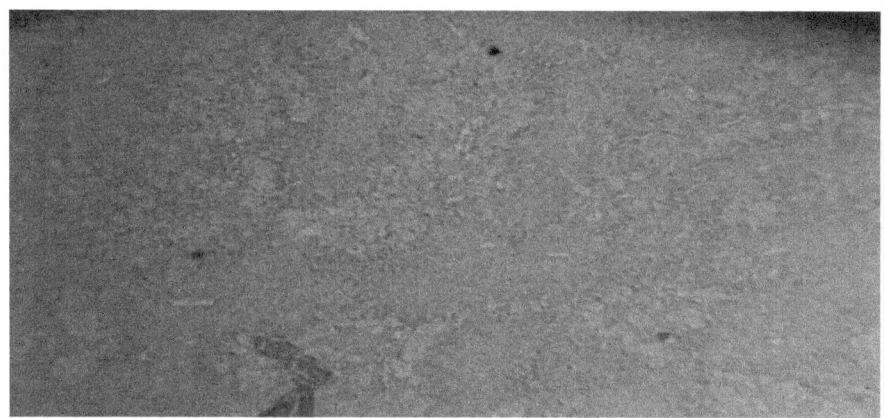

Figure (12): Acetaminophen treated liver centrizonal necrosis

Figure (13): Acetaminophen treated liver with fatty changes

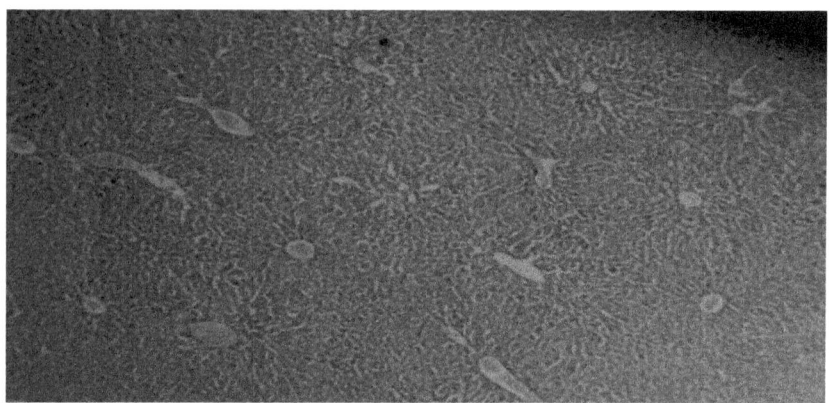

Figure (14): Ginger trated liver with no changes

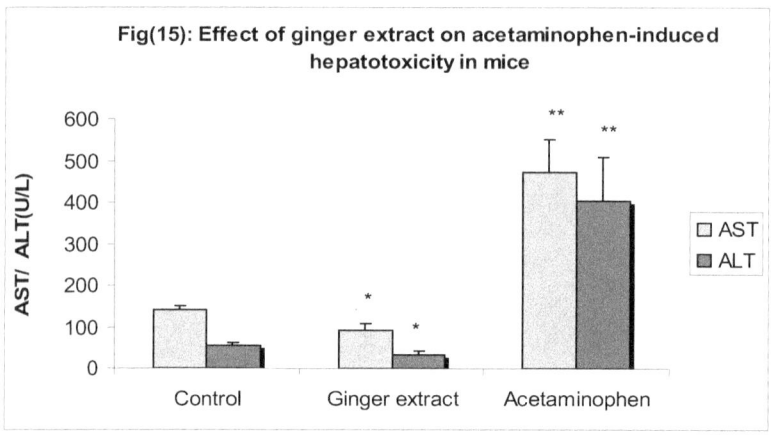

DISCUSSION: In acute parenchymal liver disease there is sudden widespread liver damage in which variable number of hepatocytes undergo necrosis. These episodes are mainly due to hepatitis virus or drug. Alanine Aminotransferase (ALT). Cytoplasmic enzyme and Aspartate Aminotransferase (AST), present both in cytoplasm and mitochondria, are the two important aminotransferases. Normal plasma contains low activities of both enzymes. ALT occur in much higher concentration in the liver than elsewhere and consequently increased in serum ALT activity reflects hepatic damage more specifically. ALT and AST are liberated into the blood whenever liver cells are damaged and increased plasma enzyme activity in sensitive index of hepatic damage. Acetaminophen causes cellular damage through induction of oxidative stress, a consequence of depletion of reduced glutathione (GSH) and significant elevation in the levels of N- acetyl – p- benzoquineimine occur, resulting in oxidative stress, cell damage and death. (Prior RL ,2003). Hepatic damage due to acetaminophen produce particularly high activities of ALT and AST 100 to 500 times the normal values. Several years ago suggested that GST formed part of a general adaptive response against cellular stress. The result of our paper indicated that (Zingiber officinale) ginger hashepatoprotective effect through antioxidant properties. (Laura PJ, et al . 2003). In support of our paper study by (.Ajith TA, et al ,. 2007). For effect of ginger on acetaminophen – induced hepatotoxicity. In this study aqueous ethanolic extract of Zingiber officinale was evaluated against single dose of acetaminophen induced (3glkg p.o) acute hepatotoxicity in rat. Administration of single dose of aqueous extract of Zingiber officinale (200 and 400 mglkg p.o) prior to acetaminophen significantly declines the activities of serum transaminase. Further hepatic oxidative status in the liver such as activities of superoxide dismutase, catalase, glutathione peroxidase and gluthione –s-transferase and levels of reduced gluthione (GSH) was enhanced in the ginger plus acetaminophen treated group than control(Omoniyi KY, Mattew CI ,. 2006).

Study of analgesic activity of Zingiber officinale (ginger) extract in mice
Hydroalcoholic extract of ginger was evaluated for its analgesic activity in albino mice, weighing 20-25g. The animals had access to water and food, but they were deprived of food 12 hour before experimentation. Mice were divided into six groups each consisting of five mice All animals were individually weighed and the doses of extract and control material were calculated accordingly. The investigation of analgesic activity by chemical method was performed by recording the number of writhes induced by i.p. injection of 0.1 ml/10 g of 1% acetic acid in mice

Group 1 : given normal saline with 0.5 % Tween-80 (1ml i.p) – ve control.

Group 2 : given acetic acid in a dose of 0.1ml/10g.

Group 3 : given hydroalcoholic extract of ginger in a dose of 150 mg /kg (i.p)

Group 4 : given hydroalcoholic extract of ginger in a dose of 300mg /kg (i.p)

Group 5 : given hydroalcoholic extract of ginger in a dose of 450mg /kg (i.p)

Group 6 : given acetylsalicylic acid in a dose of 150mg/kg (i.p) All groups (except – ve control) were injected by acetic acid 40 min after receiving different treatment. Acetic acid (i.p) caused pain sensation with constriction of abdomen, turning of trunk and extension of hind legs. This contraction of the body is termed as writhing. Any substance that has analgesic activity is supposed to reduce the number of writhes in mice within a given time and with respect to the control group. Five minutes after the administering acetic acid, the number of writhes was counted for fifteen minutes for each mouse The writhes = (The mean for every different group/control mean) ×100. Also, the percentage dose- effect of the extract on writhes was calculated as follow: Dose-effect (%) = (Total writhes per dose (T)/ Total writhes for control group (C) ×100. And the % of inhibition of writhes was calculated. % inhibition =100- (T/C×100) The values were all compared statistically with normal saline control group.

RESULTS: The analgesic effect of Zingiber officinale is shown as percentage inhibition of writhes is 51.36%, 71.36%, 77.84% and 82.5% in the animals treated with 150 mg/kg, 300 mg/kg, 450 mg/kg of zingiber officinale extract and acetylsalicylic acid respectively. The data shows that a 50% inhibition obtained at 150 mg/kg and % inhibition increase by increase the dose. By using one-way ANOVA and Post Hoc indicated that150mg/kg treated group shows highly significant decrease in the number of writhes (p0.05) compared to acetylsalicylic acid group. At dose of 450 mg/kg there was a high significant reduction (p0.05) compared to acetylsalicylic acid group. Acetylsalicylic acid cause highly significant decrease in the number of writhes (p0.05).

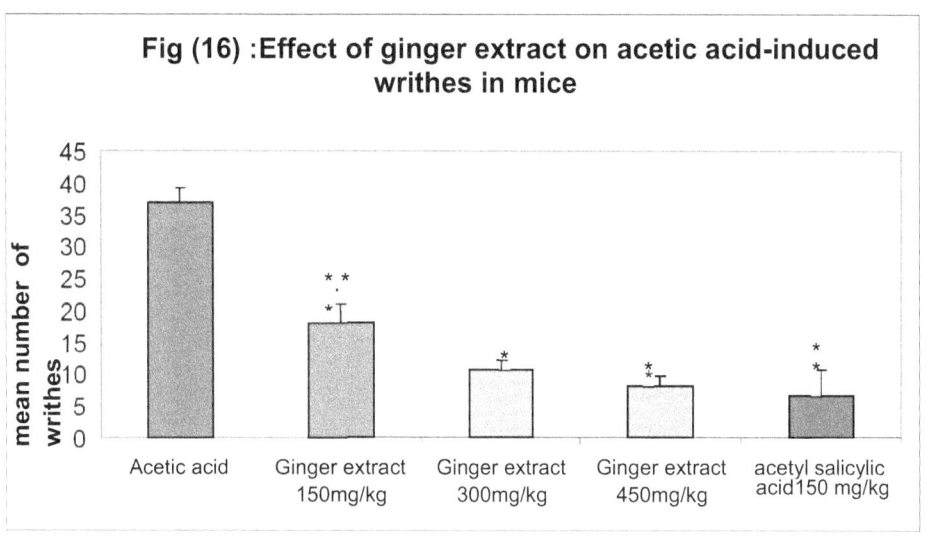

Fig (16) :Effect of ginger extract on acetic acid-induced writhes in mice

Discussion: On the basis of the common uses of this plant in traditional folk medicine the analgesic effect of the rhizome extract of Zingiber officinal was evaluated using acetic acid- induced writhing in mice. The abdominal constriction response induced by acetic acid is a sensitive procedure to establish peripherally acting analgesia. This response is thought to involve local peritoneal receptors, the nociceptive activity of acetic acid- induced writhing is due to the release of tumor necrosis factor alpha (TNF- alpha), interleukin I beta and interleukin 8 by resident peritoneal macrophage and mast cells. This is in accordance with previous studies (Onogi T et al , (1992) who demonstrated analgesic effect of Zingiber officinale extract by using acetic acid. Ginger extract in (150mg/kg, 300mg/kg, and 450mg/kg i.p) reduced the number of writhes induced by acetic acid and that the analgesic activity of the extract was increased in dose dependent pattern. methods in mice. Zingiber officinale extract (50- 800 mg/kg i.p) produced dose – dependent analgesic effect against chemically induced nociceptive pain in mice. (Young 2005) studied the analgesic activity of 6- gingerol10, which is the pungent constituent of ginger. Intraperitoneal administration of 6 – gingerol (25mg/kg- 50mg/kg) produced an inhibition of acetic acid induced writhing response and formalin – induced licking in the late phase. Furthermore, Mahmmood et al, 2004 illustrated that methanol extract of rhizome of Curcuma xantorrhiza11 (member of zingiberaceae family) showed significant analgesic activity at an oral dose of (300 mg/kg b.w) with 50.50% inhibition of acetic acid – induced writhing in mice. Whereas at a dose of (150mg/kg b.w), the extract showed moderate activity with 33.22% inhibition of acetic acid – induced writhing. The mechanism of analgesic effect of ginger is thought to be related to one of its constituents known as shagoal. This substance has inhibitory effect on the release of substance p, a neurotransmitter that is used by sensory neurons involved in perception of intense pain. Essential oils constituents such as(-) – linalool antagonize different pain response elicited by exposure to a chemical stimulus such as acetic acid –induced writhing.

References :

Ali BHG, Blunden, Tanira MO, A Nemmar (2007). Some phytochemical, pharmacological and toxicology properties of ginger (Zingiber officinale) review of recent research. Food Chem Toxicol 18: 17950516

AL-Harbi MM, Quershi S, Raza M, Ahmed MM, Afzal Ma, et al. (1997) Gastric anti-ulcer and cytoprotective effect of Commiphora Molmol in rats. J Ethanopharmacol 55:14150

Al-Yahya MA, Rafatuallah S, Mossa JS, Ageel AM, Parmar NS, et al. (1989) Gastroprotective activity of ginger in albino rats. American Journal of Chinese medicine 17 (1-2) :51-56.

Ajith TA, Hema U, Aswathy MS (2007). Zingiber officinale Roscoe prevent acetaminophen- induced acute hepatoxicity by enhancing hepatic antioxidant status. Amala Institue of Medical Sciences India. 2007.

.Barroman JA, P Feiffer GJ (1982) Cabenoxolone: Acritical analysis of its value in peptic ulcer. Drugs and peptic ulcer. Boca Raton 123-132

Goel RK, Chakrabarthy A, Sanyal AK (1985) The effect of biological variable on the anti-ulcerogenic effect of vegetable plantain banana planta Media. 2: 85-88.

Hollander D, Taranawski A, Gergely H, Zipser KD (1984) Sucralfate protection of the gastric mucosa against alcohol-induced injury: A prostaglandin-mediated process. Scand J Gastrooenterol 101: 97-102

Iranian Herbal Pharmacopea Scientific Committee (2002). Iranian Herbal Pharmacopeia. (1st edn), Iranian Ministry of Health publication, Iran 25

Langmead L, Rampton DS (2001) Herbal treatment in gastrointestinal and liver disease-benefit and danger. Aliment Pharmacol Ther 5: 12391252

Laura PJ, Philip RM, Jack AH. (2003). Acetaminphen- induced hepatotoxicity. Drug Me-tabolism and Disposition.;31(12):1499-506

Miniaiyan MA, Ghannadi A, Karimzaadeh (2006) Anti-ulcerogenic effect of ginger (rhizome of Zingiber officinale Roscoe) on cysteamine-induced duodenal ulcer in rats. 14(2): 97-101.

Mahmmood M. K, Bachar S. C, Islam M. S and Ali M. S (2004). Analgesic and Diuretic activity of Curcuma X athorrhiza; 3 (1): 66-70.

Omoniyi KY, Mattew CI (2006). Protective effects of Zingiber officinale (Zingiberaceae) against carbon tetrachloride and acetaminophen- induced hepatotoxicity in rats. Wlly Inter Science V.;20(11):997-1002.

Onogi T, Minami M, Kurraishi Y and Satoh M (1992). Capsaicin – like effect of (6)-Shogaol on substance Pcontaining primary afferents of rats: a possible mechanism of its alangesic action. Neuropharmacology; 31 (11): 1165.

Prior RL (2003). Fruit and vegetable in the prevention of cellular oxidative damage. Am J Clin Nutr.;78(3):5705-85.

.Robert A, Nezamis JE, Lancaster C, Hanchar AJ (1979) Cytoprotective by prostaglandins in rats. Prevention of gastric necrosis produced by alcohol, HCL, NaOH, Hypertonic NaCL, and thermal injury. Gastroenterology 777: 433-443

.Sakai K (1989) Effect of extract of Zingiberaceae herbs on gastric secretion in . rabbits. Chem Pharm Bull 37: 215-217

Shetty R, Kumar KV, Naidu MUR, Ratnakar KS (2000) Effect of Gingko biloboba extract on ethanol-induced gastric lesions in rats. Indian j pharmacol 32-32: 313-317.

Sertiej AA (1992). Preventive anti-ulcer activity of the rhizome extract of Zingiber officinale. Fitoterpia 63: 55-59.

Szabo S, Trier JS, Frankel PW (1981) Sulfhydryl compounds may mediate gastric cytoprotection. Science 214: 200-202.

Villegas I, LaCasa C, de La Lastra CA, Motilva V, Herreri JM, et al. (2004) Mucosal damage induced by COX-1 and COX-2 inhibitors: Role of prostaglandina and inflammatory response. Life Sci 74: 873-884.

Wallace JL (1996) NSAID gastroenteropathy: past, present, future. Can j Gastroenterol 10 451-549

Yoshikawa M, Yamaguchi S, Kunimi K, Matsuda H, Okuno Y, et al. (1992) 6-gingersulfonic acid, a new anti-ulcer principle. And ginger glycolipid A, B, C, three new monoacyldiagalactosylglycerols from Zingiberis rhizome originating in Taiwan. Chem Pharm Bull 40: 2239-2241

Young H.H, Luo Y. L. Cheng, H.Y, Hsieh. w, Liao. J.C and Peng .W.H (2005). Analgesic and anti-inflammatory activities of [6]- gingerol. Journal of Erhnopharmacology 96;1-2.207-210.

Publisher: Eliva Press SRL

Email: info@elivapress.com

Eliva Press is an independent publishing house established for the publication and dissemination of academic works all over the world. Company provides high quality and professional service for all of our authors.

Our Services:
Free of charge, open-minded, eco-friendly, innovational.

-Free standard publishing services (manuscript review, step-by-step book preparation, publication, distribution, and marketing).
-No financial risk. The author is not obliged to pay any hidden fees for publication.
-Editors. Dedicated editors will assist step by step through the projects.
-Money paid to the author for every book sold. Up to 50% royalties guaranteed.
-ISBN (International Standard Book Number). We assign a unique ISBN to every Eliva Press book.
-Digital archive storage. Books will be available online for a long time. We don't need to have a stock of our titles. No unsold copies. Eliva Press uses environment friendly print on demand technology that limits the needs of publishing business. We care about environment and share these principles with our customers.
-Cover design. Cover art is designed by a professional designer.
-Worldwide distribution. We continue expanding our distribution channels to make sure that all readers have access to our books.

www.elivapress.com